MAGNET RECOGNITION PROGRAM®

STRUCTURAL EMPOWERMENT 2023

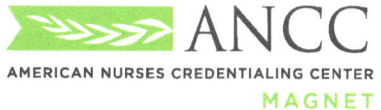

AMERICAN NURSES CREDENTIALING CENTER MAGNET RECOGNITION PROGRAM®

The American Nurses Credentialing Center (ANCC) provides people and organizations in the nursing profession with the tools they need on their journey to excellence.

ANCC recognizes healthcare organizations for nursing excellence through the Magnet Recognition Program®. ANCC is the largest and most prestigious nurse-credentialing organization in the United States.

Magnet® Program Office

The ANCC's Magnet Program Office staff manages and coordinates all aspects of the application and appraisal process.

Contact information is available at nursingworld.org/organizational-programs/magnet/contact-magnet-staff/.

For Magnet Recognition Program information online, visit: nursingworld.org/organizational-programs/magnet/

For Magnet Application Manual Updates and FAQs, visit: nursingworld.org/organizational-programs/magnet/magnet-manual-updates-and-faqs/

American Nurses Credentialing Center
A subsidiary of the American Nurses Association Enterprise
8515 Georgia Avenue, Suite 400
Silver Spring, MD 20910
ISBN-13:
Print: 978-1-953985-29-3
Epub: 978-1-953985-30-9
ePDF: 978-1-953985-31-6
Mobi: 978-1-953985-32-3

Copyright © 2021 American Nurses Credentialing Center. All rights reserved. No part of this publication may be reproduced or transmitted in any form or by any means, electronic or mechanical, including photocopy, recording, or any information storage or retrieval system, without permission of the publisher. This publication may not be translated without written permission of ANCC. For inquiries or to report unauthorized use, visit https://www.nursingworld.org/organizational-programs/magnet/.

Disclaimers:

Please note this is an abridged version of the 2023 Magnet Recognition Program Application Manual. If your organization is considering pursuing ANCC Magnet Recognition®, the Magnet Application Manual is essential for understanding the full scope of application and documentation submission requirements. It is the only authorized publication that provides detailed information on the instructions and process for documentation submission.

Completing all the processes within the *Application Manual* facilitates Magnet recognition but does not, in and of itself, guarantee achievement.

Changes may be made by the ANCC to the Magnet Recognition Program and the *Application Manual* without notice. Applicants must confirm that they are using the most current edition of the *Application Manual* before preparing written documentation for submission to the ANCC Magnet Program Office. For application information and *Application Manual* updates, go to www.nursingworld.org/organizational-programs/magnet/.

Changes to "Magnet Recognition Program®
Structural Empowerment 2023"

Page 26 Changes (continued):
  • Insert new first bullet in Note box: "SE8EO data presentation must align with the action plan described in SE7", so that it appears:

> **NOTE:**
> ▸ SE8EO data presentation *must* align with the action plan described in SE7.
> ▸ If a merger acquisition, expansion, or extenuating circumstances occur(s) within the three years prior to written documentation submission, altering the ability to meet the established goal, the organization can reestablish a goal and show progress toward the revised goal.

  • Remove words "for the two required examples" in bullet at bottom of page, so that it reads:
   ▸ A stated goal (percentage) for improvement in baccalaureate or higher degree in nursing education must be presented.

Page 34 Change: The heading "Recognition of Nursing" should appear after SE13b. and before SE14, so that it appears:

RECOGNITION OF NURSING

SE14

   a. Provide one example, with supporting evidence, of the organization's recognition of a clinical nurse(s) for their contribution(s) in addressing the strategic priorities of the organization.

Changes to "Magnet Recognition Program®
Structural Empowerment 2023"

Page 1: Insert the words: "Global Issues in Nursing & Health Care" into blue circle in "The Magnet® Model"

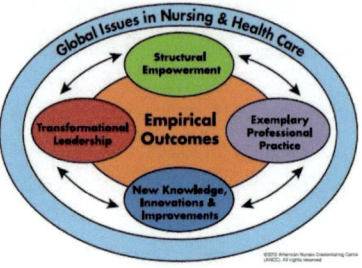

Page 20 Change: Insert new first bullet in "Note" box: SE4EO data presentation must align with the action plan described in SE3.

> **NOTE:**
> - SE4EO data presentation *must* align with the action plan described in SE3.
> - There *must* be an increase in percentage of nurses certified (only one professional board certification can be counted for each eligible nurse).
> - Present data using the required Professional Board Certification Data Display Requirements.

Page 24 Change: Insert new first bullet in Note box: "SE6EO data presentation must align with the action plan described in SE5", so that it reads:

> **NOTE:**
> - SE6EO data presentation *must* align with the action plan described in SE5.
> - There *must* be an increase in percentage of nurses certified (only one professional board certification can be counted for each eligible nurse).
> - Present data using the required Professional Board Certification Data Display Requirements.

The Magnet Recognition Program® Mission and Vision

Mission: The Magnet Recognition Program® will continually elevate patient care around the world in an environment where nurses, in collaboration with the interprofessional team, flourish by setting the standard for excellence through leadership, scientific discovery, and dissemination and implementation of new knowledge.

Vision: The Magnet Recognition Program will transform healthcare globally by bringing knowledge, skill, innovation, leadership, and compassion to every person, family, and community.

—*Commission on Magnet, 2020*

Contents

THE MAGNET RECOGNITION PROGRAM®
MISSION AND VISION   III

PREFACE   VII

CHAPTER 1 THE MAGNET® MODEL...................1
Statistical Foundation: The Empirical Model   2

SECTION II EMPIRICAL OUTCOMES (EO) COMPONENT ... 5
Empirical Outcome (EO) SOE Examples:
Presentation Requirements   6

SECTION IV STRUCTURAL EMPOWERMENT (SE)
COMPONENT............................13
Organizational Overview   16
Structural Empowerment   17

APPENDIX D SOURCE OF EVIDENCE (SOE) EXAMPLES—
TYPES AND WRITING GUIDANCE 37
Empirical Outcome (EO) SOE Examples   38
Source of Evidence (SOE) Examples Not Requiring
Empirical Outcome (EO) Data [also referred to as
a "non-Empirical SOE example"]   42

GLOSSARY FOR SE COMPONENT   45

REFERENCES   53

Preface

The American Nurses Credentialing Center (ANCC) and the Commission on Magnet (COM) are pleased to present the 2023 Magnet® Application Manual. This updated version (13th Edition) contains current information and instructions to guide Magnet® designated organizations as well as those considering the Journey to Magnet Excellence®.

ANCC Magnet designation is the highest credential a healthcare organization can achieve. It acknowledges the invaluable contributions of nurses in all healthcare settings and among all populations around the world. Magnet designation is an indication to **patients** and the public that these organizations have met the most stringent, evidence-based standards of nursing excellence in patient care delivery. It is a results-driven recognition that fosters nurse engagement, and the role nurses play as members of the interprofessional team to improve patient outcomes and reduce healthcare costs.

The revisions to the 2023 Magnet® Application Manual reflect evidence spanning 34 years of research and development. These revisions are driven by the improvements and progress seen in healthcare delivery systems around the world. The 2023 Manual was developed with input from subject matter experts including members of the Commission on Magnet, Magnet Program Office, and feedback from the field. Changes to the 2023 Manual clarify previous **standards**, acknowledge the importance of **diversity** of healthcare workers and patients, and expand upon standards in the context of an ever-evolving ambulatory care environment.

The Magnet Recognition Program's 2023 Mission and Vision inspire a sustained focus on patient care in interprofessional healthcare settings of excellence. The 2023 Magnet Application Manual standards continue to raise the bar for nursing with the ongoing development of new nursing knowledge and integration of evidence-based nursing practice. The value nurses bring to patient care, healthcare organizations, their communities, and the world is undeniable. Magnet designated organizations—of every size, patient-delivery setting, and in any location—examine and communicate a scientific impact on exemplary care delivery outcomes in the 21st century and beyond.

Jeanette Ives Erickson, DNP, RN, NEA-BC, FAAN
Chair, Commission on Magnet

Rebecca Graystone, MS, MBA, RN, NE-BC
Vice President, ANCC Magnet Recognition Program

Chapter 1

THE MAGNET® MODEL

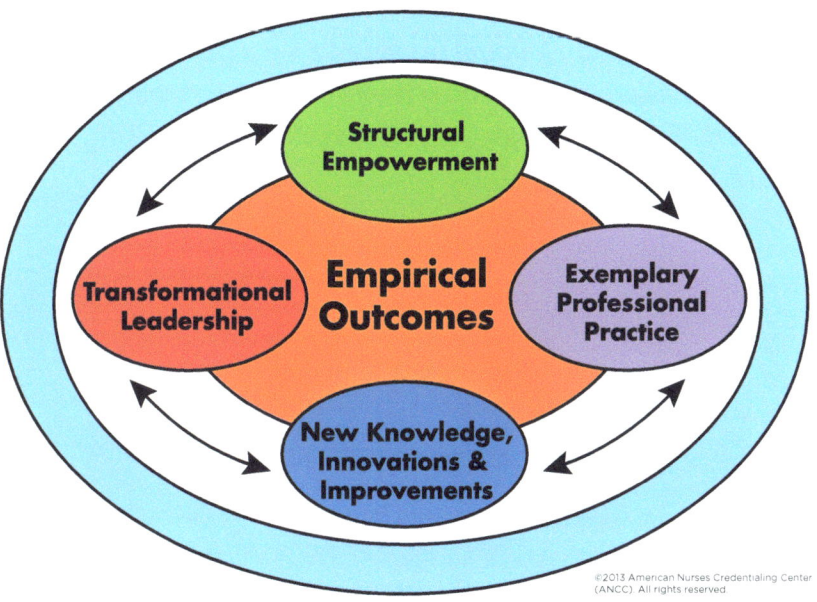

The Forces of Magnetism that were identified more than forty years ago have remained remarkably stable—a testament to their enduring value. The Magnet Recognition Program® evolved over time in response to **changes** in the healthcare environment.

Statistical Foundation: The Empirical Model

In 2007, the American Nurses Credentialing Center (ANCC) commissioned a statistical analysis of final appraisal scores for applicants under the *2005 Magnet Recognition Program Application Manual* (ANCC 2004). The project goal was to examine the relationships among the Forces of Magnetism by investigating alternative frameworks for structuring the **Source of Evidence** (SOE) examples and to inform development of the new Magnet Model. The newly developed Magnet Model first presented in the *2008 Magnet Recognition Program Application Manual* provided a new perspective on the SOE examples and how they combine to create a **work environment** that supports excellence in nursing (Figure 1.1).

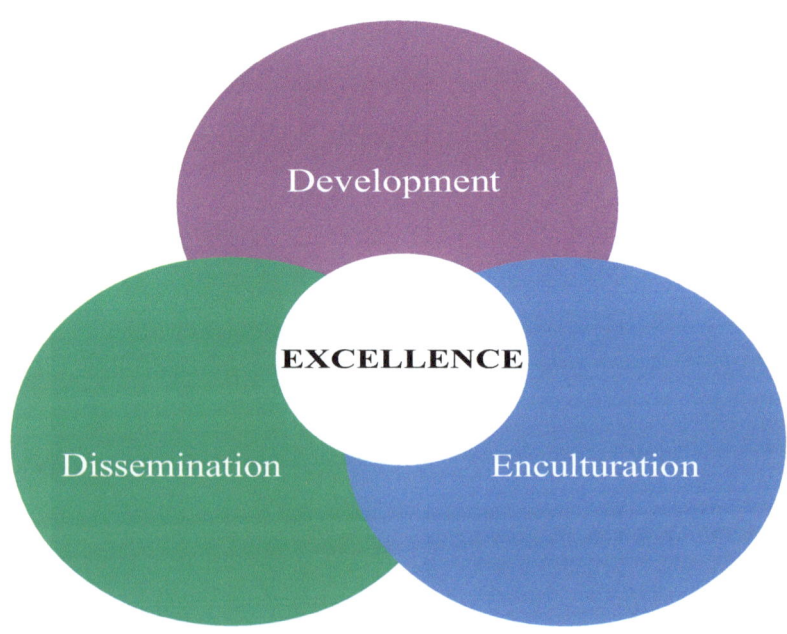

Figure 1.1. Triaxial Diagram

Through a combination of factor analysis, cluster analysis, and multidimensional scaling, the final SOE example scores were examined to determine how they might be organized based solely on their **empirical** properties. The results suggested an alternative framework for grouping the SOE examples. The empirical model yielded from this analysis informed the conceptual development of the current Magnet Model. Over the years, each subsequent manual has used a rigorous process, resulting in Magnet organizations creating a continued culture of excellence and **innovation** in nursing.

Excellence is determined through the evaluation of SOE examples, which demonstrate the infrastructure for excellence. The examples, provided by Magnet organizations, incorporate **narratives** to describe the **structure** and **process** used to achieve improved **outcomes.** These narratives demonstrate how the structures and processes are present and operationalized within the **organization**.

Before the *2019 Magnet Application Manual* was published, the **Magnet Program Office (MPO)** conducted an extensive evaluation of the characteristics of documentation submitted for review that met the threshold to move to the Site Visit Phase. The results indicated organizations that consistently demonstrated the development, dissemination, and **enculturation** of the Magnet Model Components in their documentation were the most successful. This finding established the expectation—for Initial Applicants and Magnet designated organizations alike—that the SOE example narratives and supporting evidence presented in an organization's documentation reflect enculturation of Magnet Component SOE requirements in their entirety across the depth and breadth of the organization, wherever nursing is practiced.

The 2023 Magnet Application Manual embraces the foundation set by the original study and ensuing Magnet manuals while acknowledging the importance of **diversity**, equity, inclusion and well-being of healthcare workers, patients, and communities; expands upon standards in the context of an ever-evolving ambulatory care environment; and raises the bar for nursing with the ongoing development of new nursing knowledge and the integration of evidence-based nursing practice.

Section II

EMPIRICAL OUTCOMES (EO) COMPONENT

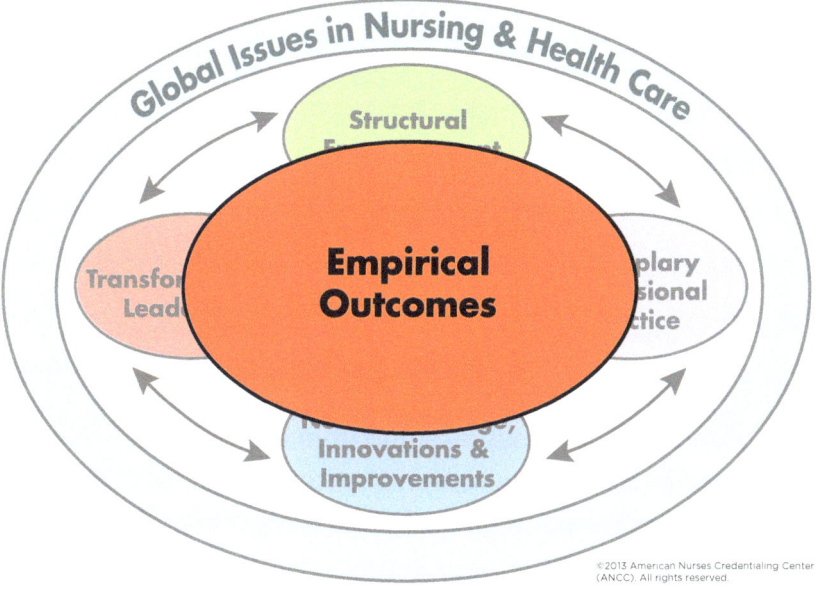

Professional nursing makes essential contributions to patient care, nursing workforce, organizational, healthcare, and consumer outcomes. The **empirical** measurement of quality **outcomes** related to nursing leadership and **clinical practice** in Magnet designated organizations is imperative. The 2008 introduction of the Magnet Model to incorporate outcomes represented a fundamental shift for the Magnet Recognition Program with the addition of the third component of Donabedian's Model of Quality—structure, process, and outcome. Previous Magnet Application Manuals emphasized **structure** and **process** and, although structure and process create the infrastructure for excellence in Magnet designated healthcare organizations, the impact of that infrastructure—outcomes—is essential to a culture of excellence and innovation. Outcomes demonstrate the achievement of desired results that are based on the healthcare team's application of sound structure and processes that exist within the organization and its systems of care.

Required Empirical Outcome (EO) Source of Evidence (SOE) examples are integrated throughout the Magnet Model Components in this Application Manual. Section II establishes the requirements for formatting narratives, graphs, and data tables, for the EO SOE examples.

Empirical Outcome (EO) SOE Examples: Presentation Requirements

Displaying data using graphs and data tables is an excellent way to illustrate outcomes resulting from the healthcare team's application of sound structure and process measures; therefore, a graph with corresponding data table (supporting evidence) is required for each EO SOE.

There are **unique EO SOE examples** that are identified in the bulleted list below that must be presented in specific formats. Specific presentation requirements for these unique examples are depicted within their respective EO SOE examples and located in the 2023 Magnet Application Manual on the page number(s) noted below.

- Page 40: Professional board certification (SE4EO)
- Page 41: Professional board certification (SE6EO)
- Page 45: Nursing education (SE8EO)
- Page 57: Registered nurse satisfaction/registered nurse engagement (EP3EO)
- Page 65: Nurse turnover rate (EP12EO)
- Page 69: Nurse-sensitive clinical quality indicators (EP19EO)
- Page 71: Nurse-sensitive clinical quality indicators (EP20EO)
- Page 74: Patient experience (EP21EO)
- Page 77: Patient experience (EP22EO)

All other EO SOE examples must be presented using the following Empirical Outcomes Presentation Requirements:

When using the empirical outcomes format, the example provided must have occurred within the 48 months prior to documentation submission.

PROBLEM

Describe the identified problem that exist(s) in the applicant organization that you worked to improve.

> **NOTE:*** The problem, pre-intervention(s), goal, intervention(s), and outcome *must* align.

> **Analysts' tip:** The outcome data drive the problem statement.

PRE-INTERVENTION

Describe the pre-intervention outcome data that drove the goal and initiative (must have occurred within the 48 months prior to documentation submission).

Describe the actions/activities that took place prior to the implementation of the intervention(s).

Include the timeline of dates of the actions/activities and the names of the key individual(s) involved.

GOAL STATEMENT

Provide the goal statement.

Include the outcome measure that aligns with the goal to demonstrate the improvement(s).

Include the location of the desired improvement.

> **Analysts' tip:** The stated goal *must* align with the graphed outcome data.

---

* Information in NOTES is very important as it conveys a requirement and/or directive.

PARTICIPANTS

▸ List participants involved in the pre-intervention and intervention activities or initiative.

▸ Include name, discipline, job title, and department.

INTERVENTION

▸ Describe the actions/activities that took place to facilitate the change and that had an impact on the problem to result in the achievement of the improvement/outcome.

▸ Include the timeline of dates of the actions/activities and the names of the key individual(s) involved.

▸ Include where and when the intervention(s) occurred (e.g., unit, department, service line, organization).

▸ Include a description of how the intervention(s) impacted the outcome.

▸ Provide key references (minimum of two) to support the interventions were evidence-based.

> **NOTE:** American Psychological Association (APA) format should be followed.

OUTCOME

▸ Provide **trended data** (i.e., a minimum of one pre-intervention data point and three post-intervention data points) demonstrating an improved trend.

- Pre-intervention and post-intervention data must be displayed to indicate the impact of an intervention or series of interventions on the outcome.

- The trended data must be displayed as a graph and table with data elements clearly provided.

> **NOTE:** The data point immediately prior to the intervention period cannot be zero.

Analysts' tip: See glossary for the full definition of *outcome*.

DATA DISPLAY REQUIREMENTS

- The graph must include dates, location of data collection, legend, and title.

- Indicate on the graph the pre-intervention, intervention, and post-intervention timeframes.

- The *x*-axis units-of-time must be the same for pre-intervention and post-intervention data (e.g., quarters, months).

- The *y*-axis units of measure represent the desired outcome. Data must be presented as ratio (e.g., rates, percentiles, percentages). Additionally, the data must be consistent throughout the data collection period.

- If data are presented for a fiscal year, the period defining the fiscal year must be defined with calendar year equivalent (January to December and year; June to May and year).

▸ Pre-Intervention and Post-Intervention timelines must be consecutive and consistent (e.g., days to days, months to months, quarters to quarters, etc.) or time intervals that are consistent with established *performance improvement methodologies*.

▸ The Pre-Intervention, Intervention, and Post-Intervention periods may not intersect.

Analysts' tip: Align the timelines in the narrative and the improvements (outcomes) displayed on the graph.

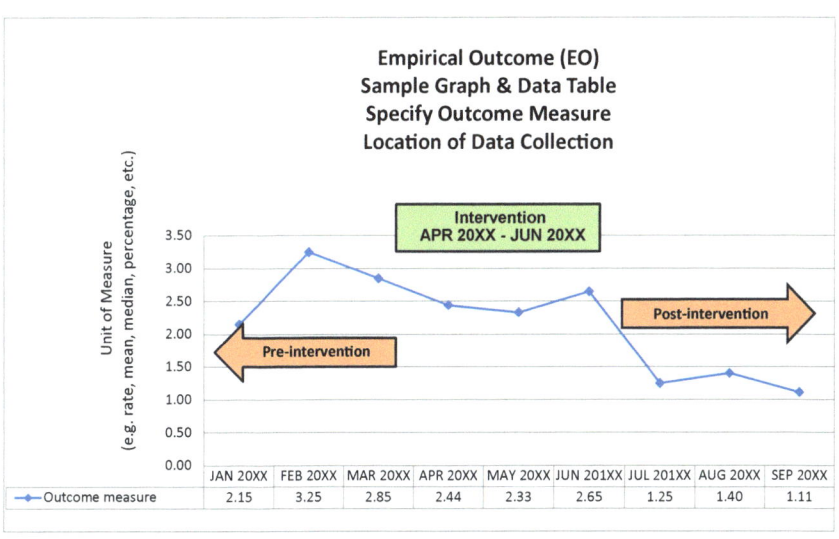

Figure II.1. Empirical Outcomes (EO) Sample Graph and Data Table

Section IV

STRUCTURAL EMPOWERMENT (SE) COMPONENT

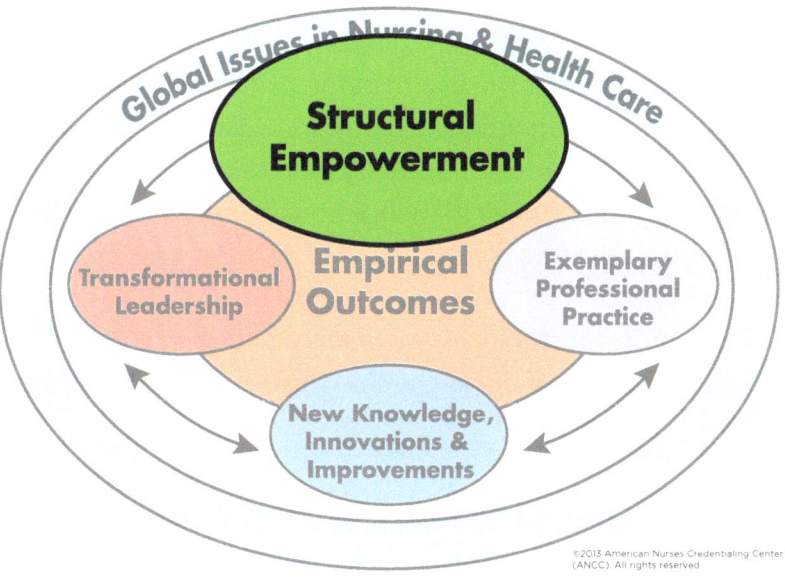

Magnet® structural environments are generally flat, flexible, and decentralized. Nurses throughout the organization are involved in shared-governance, decision-making structures and processes that establish **standards of practice*** and address opportunities for improvement.

---

* *This formatting indicates that these words and phrases are defined in the Glossary. Please refer to the Glossary for full explanations of these terms.*

The flow of information and decision-making are multidirectional among professional nurses at the bedside, leadership, interprofessional teams, and the Chief Nursing Officer (CNO). The CNO serves on the highest-level decision-making bodies, such as councils, committees, and task forces that influence the organization's mission, vision, values, and strategic goals. In addition, executive nurse leaders throughout the organization serve on decision-making bodies that address excellence in patient care and the safe, efficient, and effective operation of the organization.

Magnet designated organizations promote and develop strong partnerships with community organizations to improve patient outcomes and advance the health of the communities they serve. In addition, Magnet nurses support organizational goals, advance the nursing profession, and enhance professional development by extending their influence on professional and community groups. Nursing contributions to improve community healthcare services are acknowledged by Magnet designated organizations in substantive ways that enhance and support the value and image of nursing within the organization and the community at large.

Magnet designated organizations use multiple strategies to create structures and processes that support a lifelong learning culture that includes professional **collaboration** and the promotion of role development, academic achievement, and career advancement.

The intent of the Structural Empowerment (SE) Component is to reflect the following:

- Clinical nurses are involved in interprofessional decision-making groups at the organizational level.

- The healthcare organization supports nurses' participation in local, regional, national, or international **professional organizations**.

- The organization supports nurses' continuous professional development.

- Professional development activities are designed to improve the professional practice of nursing or patient outcomes, or both.

- Nursing continuing education assessments and implementation plans are conducted to improve nursing knowledge and impact patient outcomes.

- The organization facilitates the effective transition of registered nurses to include **new graduates**, newly hired nurses, nurse transfers within the organization, Nurse Managers, and APRNs into the work environment.

- The organization supports nurses' participation in local, regional, community, or global healthcare outreach.

- Nurses are aware of the needs of their diverse populations and deliver **culturally and/or socially sensitive care** in both the inpatient and ambulatory settings.

- Nurses in both the inpatient and ambulatory settings are recognized for their contributions in addressing the strategic priorities of the organization.

- Nurses participate in and are recognized for their contributions in interprofessional group(s) that influence the clinical care of patients.

Organizational Overview

The Organizational Overview (OO) items contain requests for documents and information that are foundational to Magnet® designated organizations and provide background information that informs the Magnet® Appraisers about the enculturation of the Magnet Components throughout the organization.

Structural Empowerment

OO4

Provide the policies and procedures that govern and guide continuing **professional development** programs.

> **NOTE:*** Policies *must* be inclusive of registered nurses. The policies and procedures may include (but are not limited to) items such as tuition reimbursement; access to web-based education; professional board **certification**; and participation in local, regional, national, and international conferences and meetings.

OO5

Provide a description and the policies, procedures, charters, or bylaws of the organization's **shared decision-making** structure.

---

* *Information in NOTES is very important as it conveys a requirement and/or directive.*

▸ Provide a description of nursing's structural and operational relationship within the organization's shared decision-making structure.

PROFESSIONAL DEVELOPMENT

SE1EO

a. Using the required empirical outcomes (EO) presentation format, provide an example of an improved patient outcome associated with the participation of clinical nurse(s) serving as a member(s) of an organization-level interprofessional decision-making group.

AND

b. Using the required EO presentation format, provide an example, from an ambulatory care setting, of an improved patient outcome associated with the participation of clinical nurse(s) serving as a member(s) of an organization-level interprofessional decision-making group.

SE2EO

a. Using the required empirical outcomes (EO) presentation format, provide one example of an improved patient outcome associated with an evidence-based change in nursing practice that occurred due to a clinical nurse's(s') **affiliation** with a professional organization.

AND

b. Using the required EO presentation format, provide one example of an improved outcome associated with the application of nursing standards of practice implemented due to a clinical nurse's(s') participation in a nursing professional organization.

COMMITMENT TO PROFESSIONAL DEVELOPMENT

SE3

Provide a narrative description of the organization's **action plan** for registered nurses' progress toward obtaining professional board certification; narrative must include:

- State the targeted goal.

- How the target was established.

- What strategies were utilized to achieve or maintain the target.

- How the nurses are supported to achieve or maintain professional board certification.

> **NOTE:** The professional board certifications used in this example *must* be included in the Magnet Program "Accepted Professional Board Certifications in the DDCT" list, located on the Magnet website.

> **Analysts' tips:**
>
> ▸ This Source of Evidence example requires you to describe the process.
>
> ▸ This Source of Evidence example *only* asks for narrative; supporting evidence is not required.

> **NOTE:** International clients may use **nursing professional development** activities for registered nurses as an alternative for professional board certification. Please refer to the Magnet Recognition Program website for other international interpretations.

> **NOTE:**
> ▸ If a merger acquisition or expansion occurs within the three years prior to written documentation submission, altering the ability to meet the established goal, the organization can reestablish the goal and show progress toward the revised goal. If this has occurred, describe the circumstances which led to reestablishing the goal.
> ▸ If there have been extenuating circumstances within the organization within the three years prior to written documentation submission, the organization can re-establish a goal and show progress toward the revised goal. If this has occurred, describe the circumstances which led to reestablishing the goal.

SE4EO

Provide graphed data (displayed as a percentage) of baseline data, plus two years of data, demonstrating nursing has met or exceeded a targeted goal at the organizational level, for improvement in professional board certification.

> **NOTE:**
> - There *must* be an increase in percentage of nurses certified (only one professional board certification can be counted for each eligible nurse).
> - Present data using the required Professional Board Certification Data Display Requirements.

Analysts' tips:

- Only one professional board certification can be counted per eligible nurse.

- Include baseline data (Year One), plus two years of data demonstrating the goal was met or exceeded.

- Applicants may use a maintenance goal if the organization professional board certification rate is ≥ 51%.

SE4EO and SE6EO: Continuous Professional Development—Professional Board Certification Data Display Requirements

The tables and graphs in this section represent the required format for illustrating the following:

1. The organization has met a targeted goal for improvement in professional board certification.

2. Nursing has met a targeted goal for improvement in professional board certification by unit or division.

A graph must be labeled with date and title.

▸ A stated goal (percentage) for improvement in professional board certification must be presented for the two required examples.

▸ For each example presented, provide three years of graphed data to demonstrate the goal(s) was (were) met or exceeded.

▸ The first year represents baseline data.

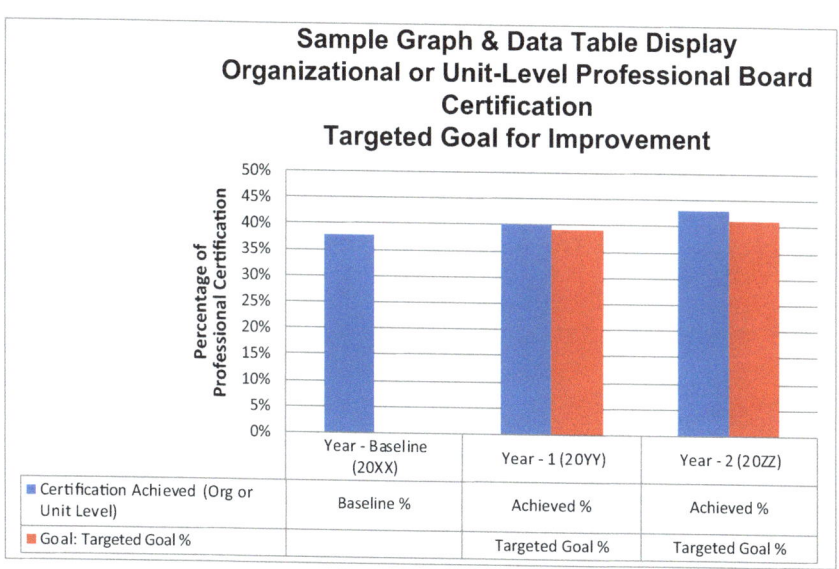

Figure IV.1. Organization (SE4EO) or Unit-Level (SE6EO) Professional Board Certification Targeted Goal for Improvement

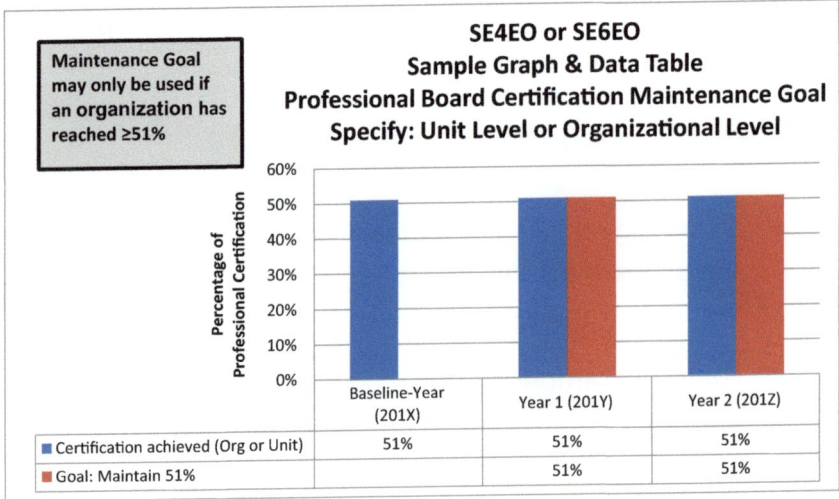

Figure IV.2. Organization-, Unit-, or Division-Level Professional Board Certification Maintenance Goal

SE5

Provide a narrative description of a unit's or division's action plan for registered nurses' progress toward obtaining professional board certification. The narrative must include the following:

▸ State the targeted goal.

▸ How the target goal was established.

▸ What strategies were utilized to achieve or maintain the target.

▸ How the nurses are supported to achieve or maintain professional board certification.

> **NOTE:**
> - If a merger acquisition or expansion occurs within the three years prior to written documentation submission, altering the ability to meet the established goal, the organization can reestablish the goal and show progress toward the revised goal. If this has occurred, describe the circumstances which led to reestablishing the goal.
> - If there have been extenuating circumstances within the organization within the three years prior to written documentation submission, the organization can reestablish a goal and show progress toward the revised goal. If this has occurred, describe the circumstances which led to reestablishing the goal.

Analysts' tips:

- This Source of Evidence example requires you to describe the process.

- This Source of Evidence example *only* asks for the narrative; supporting evidence is not required.

SE6EO

Provide graphed data (displayed as a percentage) of baseline data, plus two years of data, demonstrating nursing has met or exceeded a targeted goal(s) at the unit or division level, for improvement in professional board certification.

> **NOTE:**
> - There *must* be an increase in percentage of nurses certified (only one professional board certification can be counted for each eligible nurse).
> - Present data using the required Professional Board Certification Data Display Requirements.

Analysts' tips:

- Only one professional board certification can be counted for each eligible nurse.

- Include baseline data (year one), plus two years of data demonstrating the goal was met or exceeded.

- Applicants may use a maintenance goal if the unit's or division's professional board certification rate is ≥ 51%.

SE7

Provide a narrative description of the organization's action plan for registered nurses' progress toward obtaining a baccalaureate degree or higher degree in nursing.

Narrative description must include:

- State the targeted goal.

- How the target goal was established.

- What strategies were utilized to achieve or maintain the target (≥ 80%).

- How the nurses are supported to achieve or maintain a baccalaureate or higher degree in nursing.

> **NOTE:**
> - If a merger acquisition or expansion occurs within the three years prior to written documentation submission, altering the ability to meet the established goal, the organization can reestablish the goal and show progress toward the revised goal. If this has occurred, describe the circumstances which led to reestablishing the goal.
> - If there have been extenuating circumstances within the organization within the three years prior to written documentation submission, the organization can reestablish a goal and show progress toward the revised goal. If this has occurred, describe the circumstances which led to reestablishing the goal.

Analysts' tips:

- This Source of Evidence example requires you to describe the process.

- This Source of Evidence example *only* asks for the narrative; supporting evidence is not required.

SE8EO

Provide graphed data (displayed as a percentage) of baseline data, plus two years of data, demonstrating the organization progressing toward (or maintaining) ≥ 80% of professional registered nurses who have earned a baccalaureate or higher degree in nursing.

Analysts' tips:

- When calculating the percentage of registered nurses with a baccalaureate degree or higher, the denominator is the total *number* of registered nurses.

- The organization may use a maintenance goal if the organization is ≥ 80%.

NOTE: If a merger acquisition, expansion, or extenuating circumstances occur(s) within the three years prior to written documentation submission, altering the ability to meet the established goal, the organization can reestablish a goal and show progress toward the revised goal.

SE8EO: Baccalaureate or Higher Degree in Nursing—Professional Nursing Education Data Display Requirements

The tables and graphs in this section represent the required format for illustrating the following:

1. Nursing has met a targeted goal for improvement in baccalaureate or higher degree in nursing at the organization level.

2. Graph must be labeled with date and title.

    - A stated goal (percentage) for improvement in baccalaureate or higher degree in nursing education must be presented for the two required examples.

SE8EO
Sample Graph & Data Table
Organization Results for RNs Who Have Earned a Baccalaureate or Higher Degree in Nursing

Percentage of all RNs with baccalaureate or higher degree in nursing

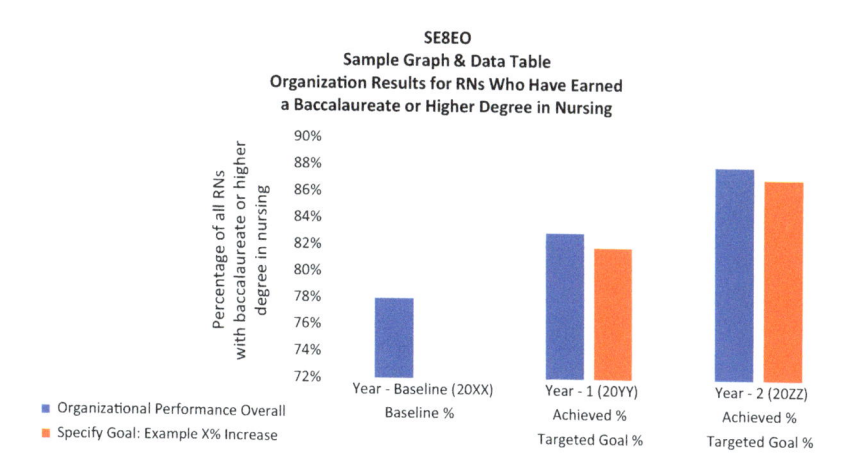

	Year - Baseline (20XX) Baseline %	Year - 1 (20YY) Achieved % Targeted Goal %	Year - 2 (20ZZ) Achieved % Targeted Goal %
Organizational Performance Overall	~78%	~83%	~87%
Specify Goal: Example X% Increase		~81%	~86%

Figure IV.3. SE8EO Example of Professional Nursing Education-Organization Results

▸ Provide three years of graphed data to demonstrate that the goal(s) was met or exceeded.

▸ The first year represents baseline data.

TEACHING AND ROLE DEVELOPMENT

SE9EO

Using the required empirical outcomes (EO) presentation format, provide an example of an improved patient outcome associated with knowledge gained from a nurse's(s') participation in a professional development activity.

> **Analysts' tip:** Professional development activities as part of transition to practice are acceptable.

SE10EO

a. Using the required empirical outcomes (EO) presentation format, provide an example of an improved patient outcome associated with a nursing **needs assessment** and a related **implementation** plan at the ambulatory care setting, unit, or division level.

> A copy of the needs assessment and implementation plan must be provided.

AND

b. Using the required empirical outcomes (EO) presentation format, provide an example of an improved patient outcome associated with a nursing needs assessment and a related implementation plan in an ambulatory care setting.

> A copy of the needs assessment and implementation plan must be provided.

Analysts' tip: The nursing needs assessment may include other disciplines.

SE11

a. Provide evidence of a nationally accredited **transition to practice program.**

Analysts' tip: A copy of the certificate awarded by the nationally accredited program is sufficient evidence to meet the standard.

OR

Select three examples; for each example, include narrative description of the five domains of the transition to practice program and evidence of quality outcomes to demonstrate the **effectiveness** of the selected transition to practice program.

> **NOTE:** The five domains of the transition to practice program *must* include **program leadership, organizational enculturation, development and design, practice-based learning,** and **quality outcomes.**

> **NOTE:** Validation of *all five* transition to practice programs will be completed during the Site Visit.

b. Provide one example, with supporting evidence, that demonstrates the effectiveness of the transition to practice program for **new graduate** nurse(s).

- Narrative must include a description of the five domains of the transition to practice program that facilitates effective transition.

- Evidence must include quality outcomes that demonstrate the effectiveness of the transition to practice program.

> **NOTE:** For each example, the narrative *must* include a description of the five domains of the transition to practice program. The *only* evidence required for each example are the quality outcomes to demonstrate the effectiveness of the selected transition to practice program.

> **Analysts' tips:**
>
> ▸ The domain of quality outcomes refers to measure(s) demonstrating the impact of the program on patients, clients, nursing residents/fellows, and the organization or practice setting(s) related to the programs.
>
> ▸ Examples can include but are not limited to **turnover rates**, retention rates, or survey results.

c. Provide one example, with supporting evidence, that demonstrates the effectiveness of the transition to practice program of a newly hired experienced nurse into the nursing practice environment.

- ▸ Narrative must include a description of the five domains of the transition to practice program that facilitates effective transition.
- ▸ Evidence must include quality outcomes that demonstrate the effectiveness of the transition to practice program.

> **NOTE:** For each example, the narrative *must* include a description of the five domains of the transition to practice program. The *only* evidence required for each example are the quality outcomes to demonstrate the effectiveness of the selected transition to practice program.

> **Analysts' tips:**
>
> ▸ The domain of quality outcomes refers to measure(s) demonstrating the impact of the program on patients, clients,

nursing residents/fellows, and the organization or practice setting(s) related to the programs.

- Examples can include but are not limited to turnover rates, retention rates, or survey results.

d. Provide one example, with supporting evidence, that demonstrates the effectiveness of the transition to practice program of a nurse transferring within the organization to a new nurse practice environment.

- Narrative must include a description of the five domains of the transition to practice program that facilitates effective transition.

- Evidence must include quality outcomes that demonstrate the effectiveness of the transition to practice program.

> **NOTE:** For each example, the narrative *must* include a description of the five domains of the transition to practice program. The *only* evidence required for each example are the quality outcomes to demonstrate the effectiveness of the selected transition to practice program.

Analysts' tips:

- The domain of quality outcomes refers to measure(s) demonstrating the impact of the program on patients, clients, nursing residents/fellows, and the organization or practice setting(s) related to the programs.

- Examples can include but are not limited to turnover rates, retention rates, or survey results.

e. Provide one example, with supporting evidence, that demonstrates the effectiveness of the transition to practice program of an APRN into the practice environment.

- ▸ Narrative must include a description of the five domains of the transition to practice program that facilitates effective transition.
- ▸ Evidence must include quality outcomes that demonstrate the effectiveness of the transition to practice program.

NOTE: For each example, the narrative *must* include a description of the five domains of the transition to practice program. The *only* evidence required for each example are the quality outcomes to demonstrate the effectiveness of the selected transition to practice program.

NOTE: Include the transition into the ambulatory provider role, if applicable.

Analysts' tips:

- ▸ The domain of quality outcomes refers to measure(s) demonstrating the impact of the program on patients, clients, nursing residents/fellows, and the organization or practice setting(s) related to the programs.

- ▸ Examples can include but are not limited to turnover rates, retention rates, or survey results.

f. Provide one example, with supporting evidence, that demonstrates the effectiveness of the transition to practice program of **Nurse Managers** into the new role.

- ▸ Narrative must include a description of the five domains of the transition to practice program that facilitates effective transition.

- ▸ Evidence must include quality outcomes that demonstrate the effectiveness of the transition to practice program.

> **NOTE:** For each example, the narrative *must* include a description of the five domains of the transition to practice program. The *only* evidence required for each example are the quality outcomes to demonstrate the effectiveness of the selected transition to practice program.

Analysts' tips:

- ▸ The domain of quality outcomes refers to measure(s) demonstrating the impact of the program on patients, clients, nursing residents/fellows, and the organization or practice setting(s) related to the programs.

- ▸ Examples can include but are not limited to turnover rates, retention rates, survey results.

COMMITMENT TO COMMUNITY INVOLVEMENT

SE12

a. Provide one example, with supporting evidence, of the organization's support of a nurse(s) who volunteer(s) in a local or regional community healthcare initiative which aligns with Healthy People 2030 or the United Nations' Sustainable Development Goals.

AND

b. Provide one example, with supporting evidence, of the organization's support of a clinical nurse(s) who **volunteer**(s) in a **population health** outreach initiative, either local or global.

RECOGNITION OF NURSING

SE13

a. Provide one example, with supporting evidence, of a nurse or group of nurses in the delivery of culturally and/or socially sensitive care.

AND

b. Provide one example, with supporting evidence, of a nurse or group of nurses delivering culturally and/or socially sensitive care in an ambulatory area.

SE14

a. Provide one example, with supporting evidence, of the organization's recognition of a clinical nurse(s) for their contribution(s) in addressing the strategic priorities of the organization.

AND

b. Provide one example, with supporting evidence, of recognition of a nurse(s) in an ambulatory care setting for their contribution(s) in addressing the strategic priorities of the organization.

SE15

Provide one example, with supporting evidence, of the organization's recognition of an interprofessional group (inclusive of nursing) for their contribution(s) in influencing the clinical care of patients.

Appendix D

SOURCE OF EVIDENCE (SOE) EXAMPLES—TYPES AND WRITING GUIDANCE

The *2023 Magnet® Application Manual* requirements are organized by Magnet Model Components, which require two general types of formatting and supporting evidence as depicted below. The Source of Evidence (SOE) examples provided in the documentation submitted by the organization should depict the Magnet characteristics embedded in and enculturated throughout the organization. Each SOE example must be clearly identified and requires a separate narrative. Descriptions of processes or programs must be accompanied by examples to illustrate how each is operationalized within the organization. The written documentation should provide examples from different departments or units to represent a variety of specialties and nursing leadership in the organization. The goal of the narratives is to clearly illustrate how the examples depict a dynamic and innovative focus on excellence as well as how they are integrated and enculturated across the organization.

Information offered for additional clarity and/or direction throughout the Magnet Application Manual is highlighted as follows:

> **Analysts' tip:** information provided to serve as guidance

> **NOTE:*** information that conveys a requirement and/or directive

Empirical Outcome (EO) SOE Examples

The EO SOE example narrative and supporting evidence must include:

- Problem

  - The identified problem that exist(s) in the applicant organization.
  - The problem, pre-intervention(s), goal, intervention(s), and outcome must align.
  - The outcome data drive the problem statement.

- Pre-Intervention

  - The pre-intervention outcome data that drove the goal and initiative
  - The actions/activities that took place prior to the implementation of the intervention(s)
  - The timeline of dates of the actions/activities
  - The names of the individual(s) involved

- Goal statement

  - The outcome measure that aligns with the goal to demonstrate the improvement(s).

---

* *Information in NOTES is very important as it conveys a requirement and/or directive.*

- The location
- Alignment with the graphed outcome data

▶ Participants

- List of participants involved in the pre-intervention and intervention activities or initiative.
- Name, discipline, job title, and department.
- A meeting sign-in sheet is not required in addition to the participant list in an EO SOE example.

▶ Intervention

- Description of the actions/activities that took place to facilitate the change and that had an impact on the problem to result in the achievement of the improvement/outcome.
- The timeline of dates of the actions/activities and the names of the key individual(s) involved.
- Where and when the intervention(s) occurred (e.g., unit, department, product line, organization).
- How the intervention(s) impacted the outcome.
- Provide key references (minimum of two) to support the interventions were evidence-based. Note: Follow American Psychological Association (APA) format.

▶ Outcome

- Trended data (i.e., a minimum of one pre-intervention data point and three post-intervention data points) demonstrating an improved trend.

- ▸▸ Pre-intervention and post-intervention data must be displayed to indicate the impact of an intervention or series of interventions on the outcome.

- ▸▸ The trended data must be displayed as a graph and table with data elements clearly provided.

- ▸ Data display requirements are also found in the 2023 Magnet Application Manual, Chapter 3, page 26.

> **IMPORTANT:** All examples and supporting evidence *must* have occurred within the 48 months prior to documentation submission. This requirement includes data presentation See Appendix C Timelines for exceptions to this requirement.

- ▸ The graphed outcome data, presented to substantiate the example narrative, represent the supporting evidence.

- ▸ Align the timelines in the narrative with the data displayed on the graph.

- ▸ Outcome data must be presented as a ratio (e.g., rate, percentage, average, mean, median) consistently throughout the data collection period. The only exception is with a "**sentinel**" or "never" event.

- ▸ A limited number of EO SOE examples require specific supporting documentation. This will be depicted in the example.

- ▸ Redact all protected health information (PHI).

Unique EO SOE Example presentations are required and depicted within the respective EO SOE examples in the 2023 Magnet Application Manual:

- Page 40: Professional board certification (SE4EO)

- Page 41: Professional board certification (SE6EO)

- Page 45: Nursing education (SE8EO)

- Page 57: Registered nurse satisfaction/registered nurse engagement (EP3EO)

- Page 65: Nurse turnover rate (EP12EO)

- Page 69: Nurse-sensitive clinical quality indicators (EP19EO)

- Page 71: Nurse-sensitive clinical quality indicators (EP20EO)

- Page 74: Patient engagement (EP21EO)

- Page 77: Patient engagement (EP22EO)

Inpatient vs. ambulatory setting examples:

- If two examples are requested (one ambulatory/one inpatient) and ambulatory settings do not exist in the organization, then two inpatient setting examples must be provided.

- If the EO SOE example request is not specific regarding the inpatient or ambulatory care setting, the example may be written about either setting.

- Ambulatory organizations that do not have any inpatient settings provide only ambulatory examples.

- Ambulatory examples must be specific to the ambulatory setting; all data must be from the ambulatory setting as well.

- Benchmarked data specific <u>only</u> to ambulatory units/areas: if a quarterly benchmark is not available, provide the available reporting timeframe (e.g., monthly, annual) to represent the equivalent of eight quarters of benchmarked data.

Source of Evidence (SOE) Examples Not Requiring Empirical Outcome (EO) Data [also referred to as a "Non-Empirical SOE example"]

The non-EO SOE examples and supporting evidence must occur within the 48-month period prior to the submission of written documentation. All protected health information (PHI) must be redacted before documentation submission.

The non-EO SOE example is written as follows:

- Narrative Statement: A description that concisely conveys how the key elements of the SOE example statement are present and operationalized within the organization. The Narrative Statement:

  - Must be a straightforward and concise description of how the SOE example is present and operationalized within the organization.

  - Must address the key words and phrases (key elements) in the SOE request statement.

  - Organizations with flat organizational structures, such as without Nurse Managers: the Nurse AVP/Nurse Director may be substituted for Nurse Manager SOE example(s).

- Example must have occurred within the 48 months prior to documentation submission.

> **IMPORTANT:** The use of the EO SOE example outline template should <u>not</u> be used when writing non-EO SOE examples.

- Supporting evidence:

  - Comprised of item(s) that support and substantiate what is stated in the narrative statements which must have occurred within the 48 months prior to documentation submission.

  - Verifies that what is stated in the narrative exists in the organization.

  - Must substantiate narrative that addresses the key words and phrases (key elements) in the SOE request statement.

  - Limit of five supporting evidence items per non-EO SOE example.

  - Acceptable supporting evidence includes (but is not limited to):

    - Copies of written policies and procedures, files, intranet sites, meeting minutes, various types of correspondence, data, rosters, committee charters, job descriptions, and screenshots.

  - To be valid, supporting evidence must:

    - Be dated;
    - Contain signatures (as applicable);
    - Be legible; and

- Include participants described in the example (e.g., name, position, title), as applicable.

▶▶ Supporting evidence does not include:

- Photographs;
- Testimonial statements; and
- Documents generated for the purpose of clarifying the narrative.

Inpatient vs. ambulatory setting examples:

▶ If the SOE example request is not specific regarding the inpatient or ambulatory care setting, the example may be written about either setting.

▶ If two examples are requested (one ambulatory/one inpatient) and the organization does not include ambulatory settings, then two inpatient setting examples must be provided. Ambulatory organizations that do not have any inpatient settings provide only ambulatory examples.

▶ SOE examples that request narrative specific to ambulatory areas must be specific to the ambulatory setting. The narrative cannot take place in both inpatient and ambulatory areas.

> **Analysts' tip:** The Magnet Program Office strongly recommends participation in the webinar Preparing a Successful Document—Critical Information. This webinar is available to applicants or members of the Magnet Learning Communities. Data indicate there is a corresponding increased success rate for organizations that view the webinar. For information, contact your regional **Magnet Program Specialist (MPS)**.

Glossary for SE Component

action plan
For Magnet purposes, a series of steps taken to achieve a goal. Action plans also typically define milestones, timelines, and progress measures and identify the responsible parties and their assignments.

affiliation
The state of being closely associated with or connected to an organization. Affiliation is the act of connecting or associating with an organization (Merriam-Webster, n.d.). For Magnet purposes, an example of a nurse affiliation with a professional organization may be as a member of a professional organization, attending a conference, webinar, or otherwise gaining information from a professional organization to improve a patient outcome.

certification
"A process by which a state regulatory body or nongovernmental agency or association certifies that an individual licensed to practice a profession has met certain predetermined standards specified by that profession for specialty practice. Its purpose is to assure various publics that an individual has mastered a body of knowledge and acquired skills in a particular specialty" (American Nurses Association, 1979, p. 67).

collaboration
"Collaboration is both a process and an outcome in which shared interest or conflict that cannot be addressed by any single

individual is addressed by key stakeholders.... The collaborative process involves a synthesis of different perspectives to better understand complex problems. A collaborative outcome is the development of integrative solutions that go beyond an individual vision to a productive resolution that could not be accomplished by any single person or organization" (Gardner, 2005, p. 1).

culturally and socially sensitive care
Culturally and socially sensitive care includes "the clinician being humble about recognizing the limits of her or his knowledge of a patient's situation, avoiding generalizing assumptions, being aware of clinicians' and patients' biases, ensuring mutual understanding through patient-centered communication, and respectfully asking open-ended questions about patients' circumstances and values when appropriate" (The American College of Obstetricians and Gynecologists, 2018).

development and design
One of five domains required by Magnet® to be included transition to practice programs (SE11). For Magnet purposes, the development domain is the process of building infrastructure, process, and competency requirements to meet a program's defined objectives, requirements, and goals (American Nurses Credentialing Center, 2020).

effectiveness
"The extent to which the goals for an activity, program, or initiative have been met" (Merriam-Webster, n.d.). For Magnet® purposes, effectiveness is assessed through the use of pre-determined outcome measures.

implementation

"The processes involved and occurring between the decision to adopt the QI [quality improvement] innovation and the routine use of the QI innovation, or the integration of a new idea or practice into the operating system of the organization" (Burns et al., 2012, p. 469).

needs assessment

"The process by which a discrepancy between what is desired and what exists is identified. This process pinpoints the level of educational intervention that is required and facilitates purposeful educational design to close the identified gap" (American Nurses Credentialing Center, 2015).

new graduate

A nurse who has completed his or her nursing education and is in the first year of employment as a registered or licensed professional nurse. New graduates are generally novice nurses who have limited clinical experience and require orientation, guidance, mentorship, and safe learning environments to transition into beginning nursing practice (adapted from Benner et al., 2009).

Nurse Manager

Registered nurses with the accountability and supervision of all registered nurses and other healthcare providers who deliver nursing care in an inpatient or ambulatory care setting. The Nurse Manager is typically responsible for recruitment and retention, performance review, and professional development; is involved in the budget formulation process and quality outcomes; and helps plan for, organize, and lead the delivery of nursing care for a designated patient care area. The title "Nurse Manager" reflects the function of the role for the purpose of documentation submission. It is understood that registered nurses who function in a Nurse Manager role in the organization may not be assigned the title of Nurse Manager.

nursing professional development
"A vital phase of lifelong learning in which nurses engage to develop and maintain competence, enhance professional nursing practice, and support achievement of career goals. Nursing professional development practice is a specialty that facilitates the lifelong learning and development activities of nurses aimed at influencing the actualization of professional growth and role competence and proficiency" (American Nurses Association and National Nursing Staff Development Organization, 2010, p. 1). See also *professional development*.

organizational enculturation
One of five domains required by Magnet® to be included in transition to practice programs (SE11). The organizational enculturation domain is the process by which participants are assimilated into the culture, practices, and values of an organization or practice setting(s) (American Nurses Credentialing Center, 2020).

population health
"The health outcomes of a group of individuals, including the distribution of such outcomes within the group" (Kindig & Stoddart, 2003, p. 381). More recently, population health has been described as "measuring and optimizing the health of groups and in so doing embraces the full range of determinants of health, including healthcare delivery" (Gourevitch, 2014, p. 544).

practice-based learning
One of five domains required by Magnet® to be included in transition to practice programs (SE11). The practice-based learning

domain is learning that takes place in the workplace setting under the guidance of **preceptors**, **mentors**, or other experienced healthcare professionals, or a combination thereof, and promotes the process of investigating and evaluating professional practices in the context of best-available evidence to continuously improve **outcomes** (American Nurses Credentialing Center, 2020).

professional development
"The activities, such as continuing education, advanced work practice, professional association involvement, teaching, and volunteer work, that credentialed professionals engage in to receive credit for the purpose of maintaining continuing competence and renewing a credential" (Institute for Credentialing Excellence, 2020, p. 15). See also *nursing professional development*.

Additionally, one of seven optional Magnet® categories for registered nurse satisfaction/registered nurse engagement benchmarking. This survey category must include a minimum of two pre-approved questions that reference education and resources.

professional organizations
"An organization whose members share a professional status, created to deal with issues of concern to the professional group or groups involved" (Mosby, 2017). "Sometimes referred to as a professional association or professional body, [it] exists to advance a particular profession, support the interests of people working in that profession and serve the public good. It facilitates innovation, communication, and connection. A professional organization typically requires member dues, has an elected leadership body, and includes a range of subcommittees or functional areas. Professional organizations can be both national

or international, and often have close ties to colleges and universities with degree programs in that field" (Indeed, 2020). For Magnet® purposes, professional organizations set the requirements and standards of practice with the intent of advancing a profession.

program leadership
One of five domains required by Magnet® to be included in transition to practice programs (SE11). The program leadership domain refers to "the oversight of assessing, planning, implementing, and evaluating the program in adherence to program criteria" (American Nurses Credentialing Center, 2020).

quality outcomes
One of five domains required by Magnet® to be included in transition to practice programs (SE11). The quality outcomes domain refers to "measures of the overall impact of the RN Residency / RN or APRN Fellowship Program on the value/benefit to patients, clients, RN residents/fellows, and the organization or practice setting(s)" (American Nurses Credentialing Center, 2020).

shared decision-making
For Magnet purposes, a dynamic partnership between leadership, nurses and other healthcare professionals that promotes collaboration, facilitates deliberation and decision making, and fosters accountability for improving patient outcomes, quality and enhancing work life (adapted from Vanderbilt University Medical Center, n.d.).

standards of practice
"Describe a competent level of nursing care as demonstrated by the critical thinking model known as the nursing process" (American Nurses Association, 2015b, p. 4).

transition to practice

"Planned, comprehensive periods of time during which registered nurses can acquire the knowledge and skills to deliver safe, quality care in a specific clinical setting" (Institute of Medicine, 2011, pp. 5–6).

turnover rates

For Magnet purposes, calculated as the number of employees who resigned, retired, expired, or were terminated, divided by the number employed during the same period. Per diem (those who float to numerous units), agency, supplemental, and travelers are <u>not included</u>.

volunteer

To volunteer is the practice of volunteering one's time or talents for charitable, educational, or other worthwhile activities, especially in one's local, regional of global community. For Magnet purposes, the volunteer activity may be a paid activity, but the activity may not be part of the individual's job description.

References

Agency for Healthcare Research and Quality (AHRQ). (2013, May). Module 4. Approaches to Quality Improvement. In *Practice Facilitation Handbook*. https://www.ahrq.gov/ncepcr/tools/pf-handbook/mod4.html

Agency for Healthcare Research and Quality. (2014, June). Chapter 2. What Is Care Coordination? In *Care Coordination Measures Atlas Update*. https://www.ahrq.gov/ncepcr/care/coordination/atlas/chapter2.html

Agency for Healthcare Research and Quality. (2018, February). *Ambulatory Care*. https://www.ahrq.gov/patient-safety/settings/ambulatory/tools.html

Agency for Healthcare Research and Quality. (2020, March). Strategy 6P: Service Recovery Programs. In *The CAHPS Ambulatory Care Improvement Guide: Practical Strategies for Improving Patient Experience* (section 6). https://www.ahrq.gov/cahps/quality-improvement/improvement-guide/6-strategies-for-improving/customer-service/strategy6p-service-recovery.html

Agency for Healthcare Research and Quality. (2020, November). *AHRQ Quality Indicator Tools for Data Analytics*. https://www.ahrq.gov/data/qualityindicators/index.html

American Academy of Ambulatory Care Nursing. (n.d.). *Nurse-Sensitive Indicators*. Retrieved April 9, 2021, from https://www.aaacn.org/practice-resources/ambulatory-care/nurse-sensitive-indicators

American Association of Colleges of Nursing. (2006). *AACN Position Statement on Nursing Research*. Washington, DC: Author. https://www.aacnnursing.org/News-Information/Position-Statements-White-Papers/Nursing-Research

The American College of Obstetricians and Gynecologists. (2018, January). *Cultural sensitivity and awareness in the delivery of health care: Committee on Health Care for Underserved Women Opinion, Number 729*. ACOG.org. https://www.acog.org/clinical/clinical-guidance/committee-opinion/articles/2018/01/importance-of-social-determinants-of-health-and-cultural-awareness-in-the-delivery-of-reproductive-health-care

American Hospital Association. (2021, January). *Fast Facts on US Hospitals, 2021*. Retrieved March 29, 2021, from https://www.aha.org/statistics/fast-facts-us-hospitals

American Nurses Association. (1979). *The study of credentialing in nursing: A new approach* (Vol. I, report of the committee). Kansas City, MO: Author.

American Nurses Association. (1996). *Nursing quality indicators: Definitions and implications*. Washington, DC. Author

American Nurses Association. (2015a). *Code of ethics for nurses with interpretive statements*. Silver Spring, MD: Author.

American Nurses Association. (2015b). *Nursing: Scope and standards of practice* (3rd ed.). Silver Spring, MD: Author.

American Nurses Association. (2016). *Nursing administration: Scope and standards of practice* (2nd ed.). Silver Spring, MD. Author.

American Nurses Association. (2021). *Nursing: Scope and standards of practice* (4th ed.). Silver Spring, MD: Author.

American Nurses Association and National Nursing Staff Development Organization. (2010). *Nursing professional development: Scope and standards of practice*. Silver Spring, MD: Author.

American Nurses Credentialing Center. (2008). *Application manual: Magnet Recognition Program*. 2008. Silver Spring, MD: Author.

American Nurses Credentialing Center. (2013). *2014 Magnet® application manual*. Silver Spring, MD: Author.

American Nurses Credentialing Center. (2015). *Primary accreditation provider application manual*. Silver Spring, MD: Author.

American Nurses Credentialing Center. (2020). *2020 Application Manual: Practice Transition Accreditation Program® (PTAP)*. Silver Spring, MD: Author

Anthony, M. K. (2006). Professional Practice and Career Development. In D. L. Huber (Ed.), *Leadership and nursing care management* (3rd ed.; pp. 61–81). Philadelphia, PA: Saunders Elsevier.

Bamboo, H. R. (n.d.). *Performance review. An HR glossary for HR terms: Glossary of human resources management and employee benefit terms*. Retrieved April 11, 2021, from https://www.bamboohr.com/hr-glossary/performance-review/

Bartz, C. C. (2010). International council of nurses and person-centered care. *International Journal of Integrated Care*, *10* (Sup), e010. https://doi.org/10.5334/ijic.480

Bass, B. M., & Riggio, R. E. (2006). *Transformational leadership* (2nd ed.). Mahwah, NJ: Lawrence Erlbaum Associates, Inc.

Benner, P., Tanner, C., & Chesla, C. (2009). *Expertise in nursing practice: Caring, clinical judgment, and ethics* (2nd ed). New York: Springer Publishing.

The Beryl Institute. (n.d.). *Patient Experience 101—Overview*. Retrieved April 11, 2021, from https://www.theberylinstitute.org/page/PX101

Bowen, C. (2020, February 12). *Patient Population*. Paubox. https://www.paubox.com/blog/patient-population

Burns, L. R., Bradley, E. H., & Weiner, B. L. (2012). *Shortell and Kaluzny's health care management: Organization, design, and behavior* (6th ed.). Clifton Park, NY: Delmar Cengage Learning.

Cain, C., & Haque, S. (2008). Organizational workflow and its impact on work quality. In R. G. Hughes (ed.), *Patient safety and quality: An evidence-based handbook for nurses* (AHRQ publication no. 08-0043) (ch. 31). Rockville, MD: Agency for Healthcare Research and Quality. Retrieved from https://archive.ahrq.gov/professionals/clinicians-providers/resources/nursing/resources/nurseshdbk/index.html

Curto, C., & Martin, D. (2020). The Magnet® site visit: Going virtual in response to COVID-19. *The Journal of Nursing Administration*, *50*(11), 555–556.

D'amour, D., & Oandasan, I. (2005). Interprofessionality as the field of interprofessional practice and interprofessional education: An emerging concept. *Journal of interprofessional care*, *19*(sup1), 8–20. https://doi.org/10.1080/13561820500081604

Darby, C., Valentine, N., De Silva, A., Murray, C. J., & World Health Organization. (2003). *World Health Organization (WHO): Strategy on measuring responsiveness*. https://apps.who.int/iris/handle/10665/68703

Dearholt, S. L., & Dang, D. (2012). *Johns Hopkins Nursing Evidence-Based Practice: Models and Guidelines* (2nd ed). Indianapolis, US: Sigma Theta Tau International.

Dempsey, C., & Reilly, B. (2016). Nurse engagement: What are the contributing factors for success? *OJIN: The Online Journal of Issues in Nursing, 21*(1), 2.

DePoy, E., & Gitlin, L. (2016). *Introduction to research: Understanding and applying multiple strategies* (5th ed.). St. Louis, MO: Elsevier.

Donabedian, A. (2003). *An introduction to quality assurance in health care*. New York: Oxford University Press.

Eggenberger, T., Sherman, R. O., & Keller, K. (2014). Creating high-performance interprofessional teams. *Am Nurse Today, 9*(11), 12–14.

Epstein, R. M., & Hundert, E. M. (2002). Defining and assessing professional competence. *JAMA, 287*(2), 226–235. https://doi.org/10.1001/jama.287.2.226

Farquharson, J. M. (2004). Liability of the Nurse Manager. In T. D. Aiken, *Legal, Ethical, and Political Issues in Nursing* (2nd ed.; pp. 311–336). Philadelphia, PA: F.A. Davis Company.

Frankel, A., Haraden, C., Federico, F., & Lenoci-Edwards, J. (2017). A framework for safe, reliable, and effective care. *White paper*. Cambridge, MA: Institute for Healthcare Improvement and Safe & Reliable Healthcare.

Friedman, J. P. (Ed.). (2012). *Barron's dictionary of business and economic terms* (5th ed.) Hauppauge, NY: Barron's Educational Series, Inc.

Gardner, D. B. (2005). Ten lessons in collaboration. *Online Journal of Issues in Nursing, 10*(1), 2.

Gourevitch, M. N. (2014). Population health and the academic medical center: The time is right. *Academic Medicine, 89*(4), 544–549.

Grawitch, M. J., & Ballard, D. W. (Eds.). (2016). *The psychologically healthy workplace: Building a win-win environment for organizations and employees.* American Psychological Association. https://doi.org/10.1037/14731-000

Griffith, J. R., & White, K. R. (2002). *The well-managed healthcare organization* (5th ed). Chicago: Health Administration Press.

Grossman, S. C., & Valiga, T. M. (2005). *The new leadership challenge: Creating the future of nursing* (2nd ed). Philadelphia: F.A. Davis Co.

Helmreich, R. L. (1998). Error management as organisational strategy. In *Proceedings of the IATA Human Factors Seminar* (pp. 1–7). Bangkok, Thailand, April 20–22, 1998.

Indeed. (2020, December 27). *Q&A: What is a professional organization?*. Indeed Career Guide. https://www.indeed.com/career-advice/career-development/what-is-a-professional-organization

Institute for Credentialing Excellence. (2020). *Basic guide to credentialing terminology* (2nd ed). Institute for Credentialing Excellence. https://www.credentialingexcellence.org/

Institute of Medicine. (2000). *To err is human: Building a safety health system.* (Kohn, L. T., Corrigan, J. M., & Donaldson, M. S., Eds.). National Academies Press (US). https://doi.org/10.17226/9728

Institute of Medicine. (2001a). *Crossing the quality chasm: A new health system for the 21st century.* The National Academies Press (US). https://doi.org/10.17226/10027

Institute of Medicine. (2001b). *Envisioning the national health care quality report*. National Academy Press. https://doi.org/10.17226/10073

Institute of Medicine. (2004). *Patient safety: Achieving a new standard for care*. (Aspden, P., Corrigan, J. M., Wolcott, J., & Erickson, S. M., Eds.). National Academies Press (US). https://doi.org/10.17226/10863

Institute of Medicine. (2011). *The future of nursing: Leading change, advancing health*. National Academies Press (US).

The Joint Commission. (2017). Patient Safety Systems (PS). In *Comprehensive accreditation manual for hospitals* (pp. PS1-PS50). Oak Brook, IL: Joint Commission Resources. Retrieved from https://www.jointcommission.org/patient_safety_systems_chapter_for_the_hospital_program

Kaya, N., Turan, N., & Aydin, G. O. (2015). A concept analysis of innovation in nursing. *Procedia—Social and Behavioral Sciences, 195*, 1674–1678.

Kindig, D., & Stoddart, G. (2003). What Is Population Health? *American Journal of Public Health, 93*, 380–383.

Lake, E. T. (2002). Development of the practice environment scale of the nursing work index. *Research in Nursing & Health, 25*(3), 176–188.

Laughlin, C. B., & Witwer, S. G. (Eds.). (2019). *Core curriculum for ambulatory care nursing* (4th ed.). Pitman, NJ: American Academy of Ambulatory Care Nursing.

Magnet hospitals. Attraction and retention of professional nurses. Task Force on Nursing Practice in Hospitals. American Academy of Nursing. (1983). *American Nurses Association Publications, G-160*, i–xiv, 1–135.

Malloch, K., & Porter-O'Grady, T. (2010). *Introduction to evidence-based practice in nursing and health care.* Burlington, Massachusetts: Jones and Bartlett Learning.

Merriam-Webster. (n.d.). *Merriam-Webster.com dictionary.* Retrieved March 29, 2021, from https://www.merriam-webster.com/dictionary

Mosby. (2017). *Mosby's dictionary of medicine, nursing and health professions* (10th ed.). Cambridge, MA: Elsevier.

National Academies of Sciences, Engineering, and Medicine. (2019). *Taking action against clinician burnout: A systems approach to professional well-being.* Washington, DC: National Academies Press.

National Advisory Council on Nurse Education and Practice. (2013). *Achieving health equity through nursing workforce diversity.* https://www.hrsa.gov/sites/default/files/hrsa/advisory-committees/nursing/reports/2013-eleventhreport.pdf

National Institute for Occupational Safety and Health. (2020, September 22). *Occupational Violence.* https://www.cdc.gov/niosh/topics/violence/default.html

National Prevention Information Network. (2020, October 21). *Cultural competence in health and human services.* https://npin.cdc.gov/pages/cultural-competence

National Quality Forum. (2004). *National voluntary consensus standards for nursing-sensitive care: An initial performance measure set.* Washington, DC: National Quality Forum.

NEJM Catalyst. (2017). What is patient-centered care? *NEJM Catalyst Innovations in Care Delivery, 3*(1). https://catalyst.nejm.org/doi/full/10.1056/CAT.17.0559

Polit, D. (2010). *Statistics and Data Analysis for Nursing Research* (2nd ed.). Saratoga Springs, NY: Pearson.

Polit, D. F., & Beck, C. T. (2017). *Nursing research: Generating and assessing evidence for nursing practice* (10th ed.). Philadelphia: Wolters Kluwer Health.

Pollard, P. B., Andres, N. K., & Dobson, A. (1996). *Nursing quality indicators: Definitions and implications.* American Nurses Association.

Shortell, S. M., & Kaluzny, A. D. (2006). *Health care management: Organization design and behavior* (5th ed.). Clifton Park, NY: Thomson Delmar Learning.

Silverstein, W., & Kowalski, M. O. (2017). Adapting a professional practice model. *American Nurse Today, 12*(9), 78–83. https://www.myditialpublication.com/publication/?m=41491&i=435651&p=84&ver=html5

Titzer, J. L., & Shirey, M. R. (2013). Nurse manager succession planning: A concept analysis. *Nursing Forum, 48* (33), 155–164.

Vanderbilt University Medical Center. (n.d.). *Shared governance.* Retrieved April 11, 2021, from https://www.vumc.org/shared-governance/welcome

von Eiff, W. (2015). International benchmarking and best practice management: In search of health care and hospital excellence. *International Best Practices in Health Care Management, 17,* 223–252. https://doi.org/10.1108/S1474-823120140000017014

Weston, M. (2010). Strategies for Enhancing Autonomy and Control Over Nursing Practice. *Online Journal of Issues in Nursing, 15*(1). https://doi.org/10.3912/OJIN.Vol15No01Man02

Witmer, A., Seifer, S. D., Finocchio, L., Leslie, J., & O'Neil, E. H. (1995). Community health workers: Integral members of the health care work force. *American Journal of Public Health, 85*(8), Pt 1: 1055–1058.

World Health Organization. (2010). *Framework for action on interprofessional education and collaborative practice.* Geneva, Switzerland: Author. http://www.who.int/hrh/resources/framework_action/en/

World Health Organization. (2016, August 20). *Health promotion.* https://www.who.int/news-room/q-a-detail/health-promotion